I Pray

SOMEONE
CUT UP MY *Midgette Campbell*
QUILT

A Caregiver's Journey
with Alzheimer's

ELOIS MIDGETTE CAMPBELL

MCKINLEY BROWNE PUBLISHING

This book is dedicated to the memory of my step-father, Samuel Bruner; brothers, Mitchell Bruner and Kenneth Midgette; sister, Deanna Midgette-Pendleton; Aunt, Nancy Smith–Hammons, and cousin, Ernest Staton Sr.

Acknowledgments

Foremost, I want to acknowledge the Holy Spirit for His divine guidance to become acquainted with Joe Hight, my editor, coach, and inspirer for writing this book. Joe is an independent bookstore owner of *Best of Books* in Edmond, Oklahoma. He launched a five-week writing seminar, and I registered for the course. Because of his encouragement and with God's strength, my mother's legacy is in print.

Special thanks to my husband, Madison Campbell, and daughter, Shelly D. Barnes, for their willingness to move from Arizona to Oklahoma to allow my mother to be closer to her other children, relatives, and friends, who also shared in this caregiving ministry.

Special thanks again to Shelly for helping me with the tedious editing process of this book, and for the inside cover artwork. Thank you *little Elaine* for bringing to my remembrance of Mama's favorite foods; it was a great help.

An extra, extra thanks to all my family and friends who were *caregivers* when Mama and I both needed quiet time: Varita Brown, Brenda McMullen, Elaine Staton (Ernest Jr.), Brian and Anne Bruner (Amber and Bryan), Michael Sr. and Rochelle Bruner (Michael Jr. and Shay Bruner, Lashelle Goff), Larry and Annetta Bruner (Keisha, Chantel, Takeya, Tamia), Elaine Bruner (Autumn), DeAndre and Tempia (Darian, DeAntre), BK and Monique Bruner (Dominique and Angelique), Bobby and Cicely Pendleton (Lindsey and Mya), Henry and Dorothy Williams, Arcola Wilson-Scott.

Thanks to many other relatives and friends who visited, called, sent cards and pictures. Special thanks to our church families for their prayers and support: Victory Temple COGIC, Oklahoma City; Prayer Assembly COGIC, Phoenix, Arizona; Equator Faith Mission, Oakland, California; and Antioch Baptist Church, Tulsa, Oklahoma.

Table of Contents

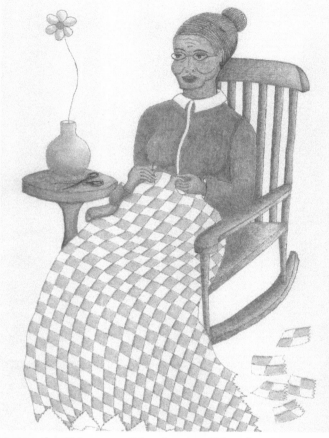

Artwork of Mama quilting by granddaughter,
Shelly Barnes.

Introduction

This book is about a disease that affects so many lives. It had an impact on me because my Mama was afflicted by it. I was her caregiver.

The national Alzheimer's Association estimates 5.3 million Americans have the disease -- 5.1 million older than 65 years of age and 200,000 younger than 65. It is said that almost two-thirds are women, and older African-Americans and Hispanics are more likely than older white people to have Alzheimer's and other forms of dementia. This is a disease that cannot be prevented or slowed down, and one in three seniors will die with Alzheimer's or other dementia. It is the sixth leading cause of death in this country.

Today, baby boomers are living longer, and every person will soon be faced with the aging process. Gerontology is a place for ministry, and the more we learn now about how to reach out to our parents and the senior adult community, the more prepared the next generation will be as caregivers of the future. The way we treat others is significant. It is evident that the best way for children to treat their parents with respect when they grow old is to train children to respect the elderly when they are young. *"Train up a child in the way he should go and when he is old he will not depart from it." (Proverbs 22:6)*

While growing up in the 1940s and 1950s, we regarded an elderly person who forgot or misplaced things as being senile or in their second childhood. We never thought of senility as anything to be embarrassed about or detrimental; it was just *old age*. In those days, most of the older people I considered senile either lived with an adult child or the adult child lived with the parents. They were family.

My mother's battle with Alzheimer's lasted at least seven years. The early onset of Alzheimer's could have been longer, but I began calculating the years from the time she lived with me and the signs were already manifesting. The title of the book *Someone Cut Up My Quilt* was the initial reason I started taking notes of my mother's extreme and unpredictable actions. I did not relate her strange behavior to Alzheimer's, or I was in denial.

Every morning after breakfast my mother would start sewing on her quilt, nothing unusual. However, one morning something was different. I thought to myself, "She is too quiet." When I entered her room a few minutes later, she was sitting in her rocking chair crying *real tears* and saying, "Someone cut up my quilt!" When I saw the cut pieces on the floor, I asked her, "Did you do that?" She said, "NO!" And I quickly defended myself and said, "I didn't do it!" I was amazed and shocked, but not angry.

This is my personal story of a mother and daughter's journey with Alzheimer's. I used Bible verses that strengthened me and might strengthen you if you are facing a similar journey. *Proverbs 23:22 says, "Hearken unto thy father that begat thee, and despise not thy mother when she is old."* These words cradled me many nights when I thought the task of being a caregiver was too much. Only God was the source of my strength.

SOMEONE CUT UP MY QUILT

A Caregiver's Journey with Alzheimer's

ELOIS MIDGETTE CAMPBELL

MCKINLEY BROWNE PUBLISHING

Mama

"Mama, I told you that three times already: You're not listening to me."

Mama repeats to me, "Where is my quilt? It was lying on my chair."

I'd reply, "Mama, you were not quilting; your material is still in your room."

Under my breath, I'm saying, "What am I missing? Why am I repeating myself?" We repeat the same statements over and over until I get the quilt out of her room and put it in her hands.

An hour later she's complaining for a different reason, "I need something to eat. I haven't eaten all day." I begin the lecture, "You ate breakfast at 8 a.m. I gave you lunch at noon. It's only 1:30 p.m." I'm mumbling to myself again, "What am I missing? Is this a joke? She's not *that* forgetful, I hope." In reality, I was definitely missing the early signs of dementia.

Before she began suffering from the early stages of Alzheimer's, Mama was our family's encourager, inspirer and mentor.

Mama, named Frankie Smith (no middle name), was born in 1920 in the cotton fields of Bristow, Oklahoma. She was the sixth child of seven children born to Frank and Minnie Smith. Mama grew up in the small town of Independence, Kansas. I remember Independence as a delightful, picture-perfect town. The town was filled with charming old homes with wraparound porches. The houses were freshly painted with well-kept lawns adorned with flowers.

As children, our special treat was visiting the Riverside Park and Zoo in Independence. The entrance into the park was as much a fairytale as the town itself. As cars entered the front entrance of the park, statues of lions captured every child's attention. The park and zoo embraced the young as well as the old with train rides, a playground, sand boxes, swing sets, slides and a swimming pool. Believe it or not, this park/zoo was there when Mama was a child. I took my daughter there, and it's still there today.

Mama's father, Frank Smith, was a masonry contractor who was well-known in the community for plastering houses; he also laid stones, blocks and bricks. Independence has a special homecoming reunion every three years to honor Independence's African-American families. At one of the homecoming reunions, my grandfather was honored. In *A Preview of Independence, KS, African-American History* by Bennie and Charlene Mosely, Chapter 7 features the "History of African-American Contractors/Builders":

> *" ... Frank Smith loved life and lived it to its fullest. He loved people and people loved him. He was a very sociable and approachable man. No doubt several houses are standing today because of the masonry skills of Frank Smith. I have no doubt that those who knew him would want to thank him for a job well done."* [1]

Until reading this article, my siblings and I had no knowledge of the sacrifices and contributions my grandfather made in this community. We appreciated Independence for sharing the legacy.

———

"Every good gift and every perfect gift is from above, and cometh down from the father of lights, ..." (James 1:17).

Mama's Early Life

My mother was a talented person. She created her own patterns to sew her clothes. She played the piano for her church, even though she never took piano lessons. Her hobbies were cooking, hairdressing, and hand-quilting, also called lap-quilting. Mama's fondness for cooking and baking started at the early age of 9. My grandmother recognized her natural gift for cooking, and soon she cooked all of the meals for the family. Her younger sister, Nancy, and niece, Elaine, were responsible for washing the pans and dishes afterward. Mama delighted in this.

Mama's parents had a vast garden planted on the north and south sides of their home. They planted wheat, corn, white potatoes, sweet potatoes, onions, carrots, tomatoes, grapes, berries, collard, turnip, and mustard greens. They also had hogs, cows, and chickens, and my grandfather enjoyed fishing and hunting rabbits. There was plenty to eat, and they shared with their neighbors. My grandfather built a slaughter-house out back to store meats, canned goods, potatoes and other food. Once I asked Mama what she'd like to do if she had enough money.

"I would like to have my own bakery shop," she said.

All of Mama's recipes were in her head or from scratch -- *a little of this, a pinch of that, a dash of this, and a shake of that, with two drops of vanilla.* Measuring cups and spoons were for people like me -- those on the clean-up committee.

Friends, neighbors, and folks from church all put in their orders for Mama's cakes and pies, such as cheesecake, coffee cake, pound cake, German chocolate cake, chocolate, coconut and banana cream pies, lemon meringue pie, and her famous sweet potato pie.

On the days Mama wanted to cook something *fast* she would bring out the rice -- broccoli with cheese and rice, Spanish rice with ground beef, beef tips and rice with gravy, and for dessert, her melt-in-your-mouth rice pudding and Rice Krispies Treats.

In the winter, Mama would make huge pots of homemade mixed-vegetable soup, homemade noodle soup in which she made her own noodles, chili bean chowder, spaghetti, hominy and ground beef stew, beef and potato stew, cabbage and neck bones, and all the greens: turnip, collard, and mustard -- all seasoned with ham hocks. She'd also prepare tuna casserole, macaroni and cheese, baked sweet potato, candied yams, homemade corn bread or hot water corn bread, and many other meats and pasta dishes.

A few of Mama's specialties were homemade rolls, fried cream-style corn, hog mog and chitterlings (a delicacy), homemade apple sauce, grilled hamburgers with a family secret ingredient, and homemade fried potatoes that were not French fries. Her all-time favorites were her handmade peanut brittle and fried pies filled with apricots and peaches.

All year long, since she was a child, Mama would preserve canned goods. She would can jellies and jams, bread and butter pickles, peaches, apples, cha-cha radish (made with pickles, cucumbers, onions, and red peppers), sweet potatoes, cucumbers, pickled pigs feet, and a few others.

My favorite dishes were cornbread dressing, crispy fried chicken cooked in a hot-grease skillet (not deep fried), fried catfish, sweet corn-on-the-cob, baked potato, grilled hamburgers, fried potatoes, mixed salad, and for dessert fried pies, cheesecake, and German chocolate cake. One or more of these dishes were on what I called *"my whenever I visited list."*

During the spring and summer months when we would come home to visit or when Mama felt the urge, she would bring out the *old* grill. It seemed as if the whole household would get up and start cleaning and singing, "Mama is going to barbecue today!" My stepfather would start mowing the yard and getting my brothers out of the bed to help. Mama would be in the kitchen preparing the hamburgers, ribs, and hot dogs ready for the grill.

If you were in the kitchen with her, you became the helper. She would say to whomever was close, "Go and get those charcoals and the lighter fluid out of the shed and put them next to the grill, so they're there when I get ready for them."

Mama had a special seasoning for her hamburgers. After adding all her ingredients into the hamburger, Mama would take some of the burger meat between her hands and press the burger lightly to form a fat ball. She never made *flat-thin* patties, but *fat-thick* ones. She would lightly press her thumb in the middle of the burger to make sure it stayed fat and firm, and not release too much juice out of the meat when grilling. The hamburgers were served with baked beans, potato salad, a mixed-green salad, and corn-on-the-cob with melted butter and, of course, a dash of salt! Also, we'd have potato chips, soda pop, and watermelon on the side.

———

"Behold, how good and how pleasant it is for brethren to dwell together in unity!"
(Psalms 133:1).

Mama's Added Responsibilities

The 1930s were the years of the Great Depression, the Dust Bowl, and job losses for many in Oklahoma and Kansas. Mama recalled buying a beautiful dress for 10 cents, which usually would have cost a dollar or more. During these years, Mama adored her two older sisters, Hazel and Izene, but both died of pneumonia within months of each other. They left between them three small children: Elaine, Sammy, and Henry -- all younger than 5. The children's fathers agreed my grandparents could provide a more stable and permanent home for them.

Mama became a mother figure to her niece and nephews at the age of 12. Many times, while sitting around and talking about the *old days,* she revealed to me that if the younger children were sick, she would have to stay home from school and take care of them. Mama's schoolteacher heard about her situation at home and sent homework to her so that she would not fail; she was very grateful to him. But life became even tougher during those Depression years. Mama and her younger sister, Nancy, had to decide who would quit high school and stay home to take care of the household, since my grandparents had to work outside the home. Of course, being the oldest, Mama knew she would be the one to stay home. She was upset for awhile because it was her senior year, but during the Depression, education was not a priority. Mama knew what she had to do and did it.

———

"...Weeping may endure for a night, but joy cometh in the morning." (Psalms 30:5).

Mama Gets Married

In 1941, my mother married my father Elgie Midgette. My dad, who was born in Haskell, Oklahoma, spent most of his childhood between small rural areas in Oklahoma and Kansas. He found work in Tulsa, Oklahoma, and they had to move.

My brother Kenneth was born in 1942, I was born in 1943, and my sister Deanna in 1945.

The marriage started out well, but *"... the trials of faith ..." (I Peter 1:7)* came to test their strength. My father was a good-hearted person. He worked for a terrazzo floor company, and the job paid well. The pay was enough to buy a newly built home in north Tulsa. But my dad was materialistic and liked to show off to his friends. If the neighbors bought a new car, my dad did the same. If a neighbor bought a new television, we bought one, too. Of course, his three children were not complaining, because we were the ones informing my dad of what everybody else had.

We lived the life of Riley and loved it. But we

needed to learn our lessons as *Colossians 3:2*
tells us, *"Set your affection on things above, not
on things on the earth."*

Mama's Silent Sit-In

After moving to Tulsa in 1942, Mama decided to take a bus downtown just to look around. At that time, she only had one child, my brother Kenneth, who was about four months old. She went into Kress, a department store, and later decided to eat lunch and sat at the lunch counter on the first floor.

Moments later, a black woman approached Mama.

"You're not from Tulsa, are you?"

"No," Mama said.

"Well you probably don't know this, but all colored people are only served downstairs."

Mama said, "Oh, OK" and followed the woman downstairs. When she looked around and saw the dirty counters, filthy tables and chairs, she politely told the woman, "I'm not eating down here. I'm going back upstairs!" Mama turned and went back up the stairs. When Mama was at the upstairs lunch counter again, her same seat was still vacant. Mama sat down,

and the waitress came over and waited on her
without mumbling a word.

I always teased her about being the first
black demonstrator without encountering a
riot. Mama reminded me of the courage of *Es-
ther 4:16 ..."I go in unto the king, which is not
according to the law; and if I perish, I perish."*

Mama certainly knew about prejudice, but
was never intimidated by other people's prej-
udices. She had always attended integrated
school in Independence, Kansas, since 1925.
Blacks and whites shopped at the same stores,
played in the same park, and walked the streets
together without any trouble. Therefore, sitting
at a lunch counter in Tulsa in 1942 was natural
for her.

When she was young, Mama's best friend
was a white girl. However, as they got older, the
girl told her that they couldn't speak or play together on the weekends, but had to wait until
they were at school. Mama told her that she understood. Mama truly felt sorry for her friend,
because on the weekends her other white class-
mates had nothing to do with her. The girl told

Mama secretly that she always looked forward to school, because she could talk and share with Mama, her only friend.

———

"A man that hath friends must show himself friendly: and there is a friend that sticketh closer than a brother." (Proverbs 18:24).

Mama Faces More Challenges

One morning in 1945, when I was 2½ years old, Mama called out to me to come to the kitchen.

I yelled back, "I can't!"

She repeated again for me to come to her.

Again I yelled, "I can't!"

Then she came to me and picked me up off the bed. She stood me on the floor, and my legs collapsed like a rubber band. Mama screamed, "Call Dr. Bryant!" In those days, some doctors made house calls.

The doctor told Mama I had contracted polio. In the 1940s, many cases of polio were being reported. There was no specialist or therapy clinic in Tulsa that could treat polio, so Dr. Bryant referred Mama to an Oklahoma City doctor. We soon were taking a train once a week for about six months to visit the therapist.

Mama related to me an incident she had with a nurse on our first day at the doctor's office. The receptionist checked us in, and we waited to be called into his office. When the nurse called Mama to enter, she quickly stated, "The doctor does not see COLORED people!" Mama politely said, "I was referred to him by my doctor in Tulsa. I took a train, paid a taxi driver to get here, and you're telling me I can't see the doctor." At that time, the doctor -- I never knew his name -- heard the conversation and stamped out of his office.

"Don't you ever speak to MY patient in that *tone* of voice again, and never *assume* that I do not receive COLORED people," he yelled at the nurse.

We continued my therapy for six months, and Mama said she never saw that nurse again. Whether fired or not, she was never in the office on the days we were scheduled to visit.

On the days that Mama had to take me to Oklahoma City for therapy, her mother would take a train from Independence, Kansas, to baby-sit my 3-year-old brother, Kenneth, and my 6-month-old sister, Deanna, while my father worked.

My therapy had to be on-going when at

home. Mama would have to massage my legs at least three or four times a day to keep the muscles from cramping. She trained my father and brother how to massage my legs when she was tired. One day, Mama fell asleep while my brother was massaging my legs. He kept trying to wake her up. Finally he said, "Mama, Mama, I'm tired of rubbing Elois's legs. I wanna go to sleep, too!"

Every morning Mama always turned on the radio, not only for herself but because I also liked listening to music. On one particular morning, a fast-moving song came on the radio, and she heard me laughing in my room. Mama peeked around the corner and saw me dancing to the music. Without thinking, she started screaming so loud that I fell down. When she realized she had frightened me, Mama stood me back up on my feet and said, "Keep dancing, baby! Keep dancing!"

I have been dancing ever since: *"And David danced before the Lord with all his might; ..." (2 Samuel 6:14).*

Mama's faith in God kept her going when

friends could not come around, or when a
neighbor decided to pass a petition around to
the other neighbors wanting to quarantine our
house. But Mama understood, because polio
was contagious. However, the neighbors did
not sign the petition, and the health department
stepped in and declared our home safe.

Today, as I reminiscence about my mother's
battle with Alzheimer's, I ask myself, "Who am
I to complain about anything?" It was an honor
and my *reasonable service*. I cannot pay it forward to her, but I can take this time to leave a
legacy of her work to others. Mama lived a long
and prosperous life. I pray that my FAITH will
be as strong and that my life will be even more
productive and that someone will see Christ in
my life.

———

*"I beseech you therefore, brethren, by the
mercies of God, that ye present your bodies,
a living sacrifice, holy, acceptable, unto God
which is your reasonable service."*
(Romans 12:1).

Mama's Divorce

After we started school full time, Mama pursued her dream to become a beautician. After taking cosmetology courses day and night, she received her license from The Madam Walker Beauty School in Tulsa and started working as a hairdresser at home. Most of her clients were the young girls in our neighborhood, and they usually called her Aunt Frankie or Miss Frankie. Mama, knowing their parents could not pay much, was sensitive and understanding as to what she charged. If Mama's elderly clients were not physically able to come to our home, she would pack up her straightening comb and curling iron and go to their home, but only if they lived within walking distance, because she didn't drive.

The early 1950s were seemingly great years for our family, but when I was 12 I began to notice my father's drinking problems. On weekends, my parents would argue about money and how my father would hang out with the "good ole boys" on Friday nights. Instead of bringing his paycheck home, he would purposely set up drinks for the boys, showing them who was the man in his house. Finally, my father's drinking habits had to be dealt with, and my parents divorced after 16 years of marriage. Soon after, my father moved to Oakland, California. For many years until his death in 1997, my father said he regretted the foolishness of his actions.

I remember Mama keeping a positive attitude throughout the divorce. The Christmas of 1957, Mama approached the three of us children and said, "Things might get a little rough financially, but we'll make it." We prepared not to have a Christmas tree or exchange presents. In fact, we enjoyed just having peace and quiet from all the chaos that alcohol abuse can bring to a home. That Christmas Eve, Kenneth ran home and told Mama that a man in a large truck was giving away Christmas trees.

"Would it be OK to get one?"

Mama quickly replied, "Of course, go get it!"

Instead of bringing one tree home, Kenneth brought two. Mama said, "We only have enough decorations for one tree, but see if someone else in the neighborhood needs a tree and if not, you can bring it back home." Kenneth did find someone to take the other tree.

We created decorations for the tree with material and scraps of construction paper, and Mama made peanut brittle, sugar cookies, and popcorn balls. I remember thanking God for sending our family that Christmas tree, even when we all decided to do without. At that time, it was the best Christmas Eve ever!

———

"A man hath joy by the answer of his mouth ..." (Proverbs 15:23).

Life Must Go On

Mama remarried in 1959 to my stepfather, Samuel Bruner. He was a widower with three children -- Mitchell, Larry, and Elaine. Mitchell was 16 years old, Larry 7 and Elaine 5 when they married. Kenneth was 17, I was 16, and Deanna 14. Mama later gave birth to two more sons, Michael and Brian. We were now a family of eight children.

My stepfather was not a stranger to us. Mitchell, his oldest son, had been our friend since preschool. His mother would bring him over to play, so he was already like family to us. He called Mama, Aunt Frankie, and we called him our cousin. Mitchell's mother died when he was 12, and his grandmother moved into their home to take care of them. When Mitchell and I saw each other at school, we'd always say, "Hey cousin!"

Blending two families into one house was frustrating for me. We moved from a two-bedroom, one-bath home with four people into a

two-bedroom, one-bath home with eight people; however, my stepfather's house was much
larger in square footage.   My other siblings
didn't protest as much as I did. They'd say, "You
do what you have to do!" With the new sleeping
arrangements, three girls slept in one bed instead of two. Showers were taken in the laundry
room in the garage. Laundry and ironing were
the biggest chores. Before, everyone took care
of their own washing and ironing; now, Deanna
and I had assignments as to who washed, folded,
and ironed. Did my attitude disturb my mother?
Of course not, because life went on.

Mama had two stipulations for us: 1. No one
had to run away from home. And, 2. If we continued to live in her house, we would all graduate from high school.

Because Mama did not graduate from high
school, she wanted to instill in us the value of
receiving a high school diploma. Mama also told
us, especially the older kids, that she would help
us leave home, if that was our desire. I thought
FANTASTIC, my dream come true! I could do
what I wanted, get a job that paid well, get an

apartment, sleep in late, and travel. But Mama didn't want to spoil our dreams and tell us the consequences of leaving home -- that there would be no moving back in, except to visit.

Consequently, there was a lot of moving in and moving out during the '60s. Kenneth graduated from Booker T. Washington High School in Tulsa in 1960 and moved to Los Angeles. He was not the first to graduate from Booker T. I graduated in 1961 and moved to Omaha, Nebraska. Mitchell graduated in 1962 and joined the Air Force. I moved back home in 1962 and when Deanna graduated in 1963, we both moved to Oakland, California. By the end of the summer of 1963, there were only four kids at home. Mama would say to us, "You are now GROWN and on your OWN!"

Today, as I reflect back to when Mama was 12, and her two sisters died and left three small children, I also think about Mitchell losing his mother at 12. He also had two siblings to help care for, and a few years later his grandmother died. I believe Mama related to Mitchell in a special way because she knew the burden those responsibilities could have on an adolescent child.

I also believe Mama was destined to stand in the gap and become a mother to our new brothers and sister. They loved and respected her dearly, and they referred to her not as their stepmother, but as Aunt Frankie and then Mama. I saw the love they had for her and that could have been why I resented the change so much. I was possessive of my mother and did not like to share her with others. But we became a family, and Mama was the glue that kept our small clan together. Also, we never used the terms stepbrother, stepsister, or half, and no one taught us this. We just made the decision not to make a distinction between ourselves. Other people tried, but we always referred to each other as brother and sister. To be a family, we had to pull together, and we did. We needed each other. Before my stepfather died, Mama said, he congratulated her for keeping the kids together through the years.

Mama was always there for us. Whenever we had problems or wanted to complain about something, or just needed a shoulder to cry on, someone would say, "CALL MAMA!" We all knew just by hearing her voice, everything would work out. Even if we disliked her advice, Mama still had the answers.

―――――

"And we know that all things work together for good to them that love God, to them who are the called according to his purpose."
(Romans 8:28).

Family Gatherings

Whenever possible, we always tried to go to Mama's house, whether it was Thanksgiving, Christmas, a summer fish fry, a birthday party, or a family reunion. When at home, everyone enjoyed gathering in my parent's backyard, which faced the street and was shaded by two huge green trees. Some of us liked to sit in lawn chairs or on colorful blankets spread out on the grass. We would all wave and greet everybody and anybody. No one was required to know the people who passed by in their cars or that walked down the street; we would just wave and say, "How you doin'." It was Mama's way of greeting people, and we all picked up on it.

If you were a relative or friend of the family and passing through the city, Mama would insist on you spending the night. During the '50s and '60s, no one drove the highways at night; it was too dangerous and in many areas blacks were not allowed to stay in motels or hotels. Most black drivers tried to get to their destination before dark. If there was not another driver in the car, the driver would pull off the road for a quick shut-eye, no more then 20-30 minutes, and then keep moving. Even today, I do not recommend driving at night. I always advise, "Please, spend the night."

Although Mama's home had only two bed-rooms, she would find a place for guests to sleep comfortably. Both the living and family room sofas converted into beds, so everyone had somewhere to sleep, and no one ever had to sleep on the floor. When I would visit, my favorite place to sleep was on the living room sofa by the fireplace. Whether the fireplace was lit or not, it was a serene and blissful area. It was *home*.

———

"How beautiful are the feet of them that ...
bring glad tidings of good things!"
(Romans 10:15b).

Evidence of Alzheimer's

In 2002, I took a course in Gerontology at Master's Graduate School of Divinity in Evansville, Indiana. I decided to take the course because I was reaching the age of retirement and researching information that would benefit me in my golden age. I didn't realize how soon I would use that information.

My stepfather died in 1999 at the age of 87. His death was the main factor in relocating my mother to Peoria, Arizona, where I was living at the time. I, being retired, had the most time to spend with Mama than my other siblings did. I had always dreamed that when I retired, Mama and I could travel together, visit relatives out-of-state and just have a great time together. It never occurred to me that the disease of Alzheimer's would invade our lives.

My mother was always fairly healthy, but as she grew older she was hospitalized on several occasions for congestive heart failure. In 2002, Mama was hospitalized for severe intestinal bleeding and was given several pints of blood. She had coughed up blood after eating spoiled food. During the hospital stay, I began to notice that Mama was confused about certain things. She didn't remember being taken to the hospital in an ambulance. And on the day of her dismissal, I had brought her clothing from home, but when I entered her room, she was already fully dressed. She had put on her roommate's clothing, which happened to fit her perfectly, thinking they were her own. When I asked where she had gotten the clothes, she insisted they were her own. The nurse, who helped her get dressed, soon realized the clothing belonged to her roommate, who was moved to another room. The nurse was able to persuade Mama to change clothes. And I was grateful we didn't leave the hospital with the wrong clothes.

After this incident, I moved Mama to Arizona. A few months later, in January of 2003, my sister Deanna died at the age of 58 from a severe asthmatic attack in Oakland. Our family came from various places to attend Deanna's funeral. After the funeral, as our family members started to leave to travel back to their homes, Mama became agitated and wanted to return to Oklahoma. My cousin, Elaine, who lives in Oklahoma, volunteered to drive her back to Oklahoma.

After a week in Oklahoma, Mama wanted to return to Arizona. I flew to Oklahoma, picked her up and did an immediate turn-a-round back to Arizona. Three days later, Mama said, "I want to go home." I explained to her, "You just got back from home. Why do you want to go back so soon?" She didn't answer. I then realized she thought I lived around the corner and that I could just get in my car and take her back and forth. The trips to Oklahoma came to a halt.

———

"For God is not the author of confusion, but of peace ..." (I Corinthians 14:33).

Legal and Financial Affairs

A few months before I decided to move Mama from Oklahoma, I realized she needed to appoint someone to handle her personal affairs, just in case she had another medical incident. Mama, now in her 80s, did not have a problem giving my younger brother and me authorization for acquiring power of attorney. My younger brother, Michael, who lived in Oklahoma, was appointed the first person to contact, and I, being out-of-state, was appointed the second contact.

Mama always watched her finances. I gave Mama her bank statements every month, so she could review her finances. She liked to have enough money in her purse, as she would say, "Just in case I want to go home." I would give her enough cash, at least the amount she requested, to keep in her purse for her own personal assurance. I also was concerned Mama would try to leave on her own trying to return home, but I relied on this Scripture: *"Let not your heart be troubled; ye believe in God, believe also in me." (John 14:1).* I relied on this word of God, which enabled me to convince her that it was too dangerous for "older women" to travel without someone accompanying them.

Mama would count her money two to three times a day, which later became confusing and frustrating for her. So, I began to issue her $1 bills to keep in her purse. A minimum of 20 $1 bills was sufficient for her. She loved to tip people whenever they did little things for her, and having $1 bills prevented her from unknowingly tipping $20. Eventually, the money situation resolved itself when she stopped asking for the bank statements and stopped counting her money, because money became of no value to her. She stopped pulling out $1 bills and began to carry an empty black purse with a few Kleenex and napkins. Later, she never bothered to look inside the purse again, and then stopped carrying it.

————

"No man can serve two masters...Ye cannot serve God and mammon." (Matthew 6:24).

The Personalities

Mama perceived me as three different people. She would literally close her eyes, wait a minute and when she opened them, I was a totally different person. I watched Mama's facial expression change from friendly recognition of me as her daughter, the one she can trust, to a nurse who was giving her instructions and medications, which made her think she was in the hospital. The third person would be a stranger who wanted to harm her, and she needed to run away. How frightful that must be, not knowing who you are, or where you are, and asking for your mom and dad. Some say that many Alzheimer's patients who had everything may even think God has left them.

I also saw Mama's character change into three different personalities. Sometimes she was Mama and we would share things about the past, laugh a little, and it would be great. But in the twinkling of an eye, I could leave the room and return, and I'd be talking to a different per-

son. This person was argumentative and ready
to leave the house. The third person I'd encoun-
ter had a childlike mentality, and she would insist on my full, undivided attention, and *fake*
her cries when she couldn't have her way. It was
difficult to handle.

———

"... I will never leave thee, nor forsake thee."
(Hebrews 13:5).

Going to the Doctor

After moving Mama to my home, I located a primary care physician for her. After several visits, he suggested I take Mama to a neurologist for a complete evaluation and diagnoses of Alzheimer's. The neurologist asked her various questions: "What is today's date? Who is the president? Count 100 backward." I could see immediately the doctor was annoying her, and she screamed, "You think I'm crazy! Well, I'm not!" She pointed to me and said, "She is the one that is sick, not me!" Then Mama refused to answer any more of his questions, and we left his office. That was the last time we saw him. The neurologist only got enough information to diagnose her case as the onset stage of dementia.

When leaving home for any reason, whether it was the doctor's office or just a ride in the car, two items had to be in Mama's possession: her red wool coat and her black purse. Winter, spring, summer, or fall, Mama wanted to wear her red coat. So during the summer months, I substituted a red house robe for the red wool coat.

Our trips to the doctor's office were often dramatic. Just to get her to the doctor took some maneuvering on my part. I would schedule all her appointments early in the morning. She would already be up early to have coffee, and I could easily get her dressed while she waited for her coffee.

"Let's go," I'd say.

"Where are we going?"

"You have a doctor's appointment, remember!"

After getting her in the car, Mama would ask, "Why does the doctor want to see me?" Then I would tell her that Deanna, my deceased sister, was going to meet us at the doctor's office, and he would tell us all together why he wanted to see her. If she asked me about my sister's whereabouts after we arrived at the doctor's office, I would tell her that Deanna was parking her car. While talking with her doctor, Mama usually forgot about my sister. Her mind would go elsewhere, and I would thank the Lord for getting us through another doctor's visit.

Yes, I had to fabricate stories to get her to the doctor's office or to get her to go anywhere. I made stories up as I was driving. Even Christians have to do what works. *Romans 14:19 says, "Let us, therefore follow after the things which make for peace,"* and I will do and say many things for PEACE.

At times, when I had to park far from the building, I would leave Mama inside the medical building sitting in a wheelchair while I went to get the car. I always brought along her wheelchair so she could sit in it instead of having to stand.

Once, when I walked in the building after getting the car, Mama was sitting on the floor next to the wheelchair. I thought, "She could not have fallen, because the wheelchair is still locked and sitting upright, and if it had tilted over, the wheelchair would have been too heavy for her to pick up." However, there she was sitting on the floor, and I couldn't pull her up. Then I prayed two words, "JESUS HELP!" At that time, two young men got off the elevator and asked me if I needed help. I immediately said, "YES," and they picked Mama off the floor and put her into the wheelchair. On days like this, I hated doctor's appointments. But I was glad that God answers short, desperate prayers.

There were days at the doctor's office when everything went well, and there were days when I wished I stayed in bed. Then there were the days Mama refused to buckle her car seatbelt, and I would have to move her to the backseat. After coming home from the doctor's office, I'd be totally exhausted.

Everyone wants to be on their *best behavior* in public, and no one wants to be accused of elder abuse. At times, when trying to help Mama out of the wheelchair, I'd take her by the arm or move her feet to stand up, and if she had an audience, she cried out, "You're hurting me!" If no one was around, she was quiet as a lamb and sweet as a hummingbird, but if someone was visible, the SHOW WAS ON!

Did I complain, sure I did, but thank the Lord for Psalms 27:14 *"Wait on the Lord: and be of good courage, and he shall strengthen thine heart: Wait, I say, on the LORD."* I was learning the servitude role in caregiving.

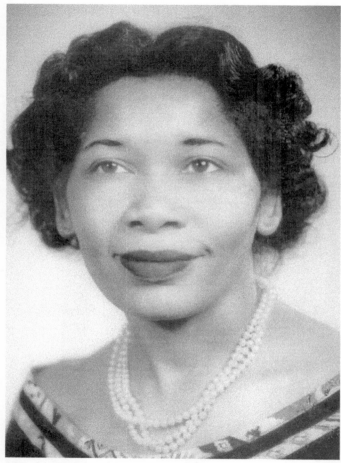

Frankie Smith Midgette Bruner.

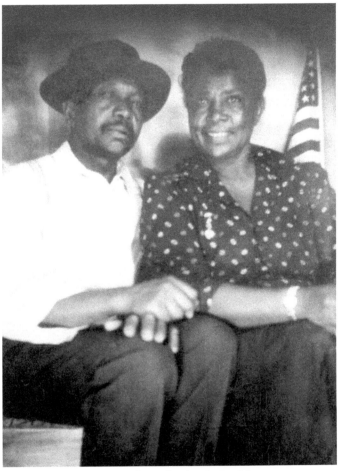

Mama's parents, Frank and Minnie Smith.

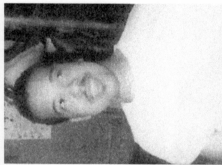
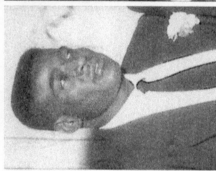
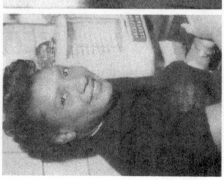

Mama's sister Hazel's children, niece Elaine Ford and Sammy Jr. Ford and her sister Izene's son, Henry Williams.

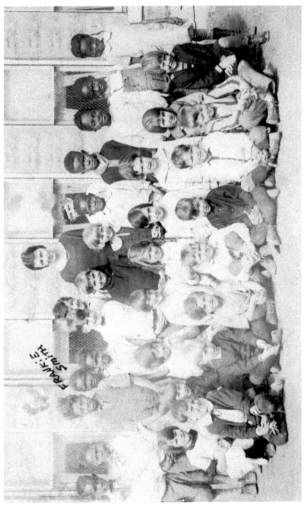

1928-1929 McKinley Elementary School in Independence, Kansas: Mama's grade-school class.

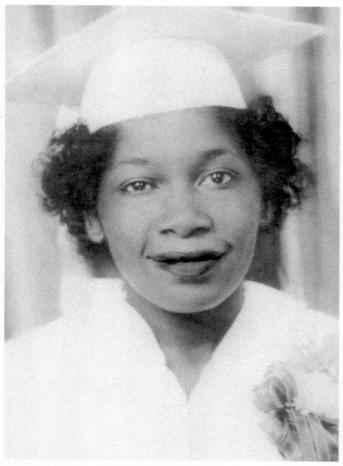

Mama graduated from Madame Walker Beauty College, Tulsa, Oklahoma in 1950.

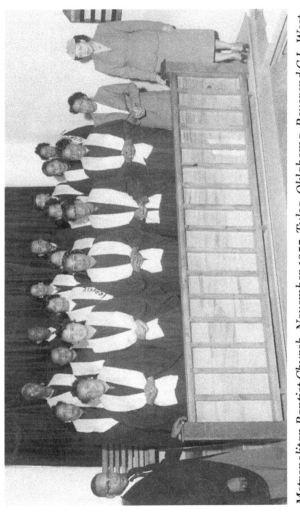

Metropolitan Baptist Church, November 1955, Tulsa, Oklahoma, Reverend C.L. West was pastor. Mama and Aunt Nancy sang in the choir. This is the church where I grew up and played the piano for the youth choir.

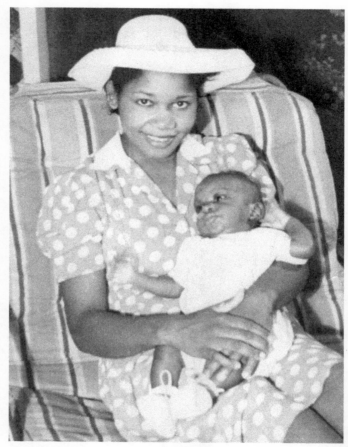

Mama Frankie with her oldest children, Kenneth, 1942.

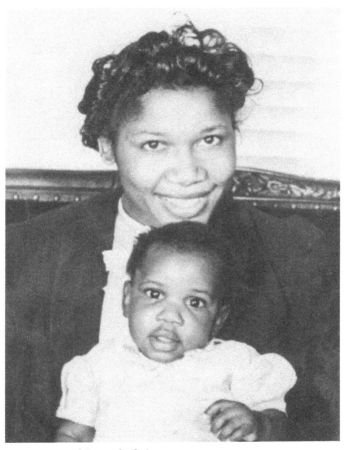

Mama Frankie and Elois, 1943.

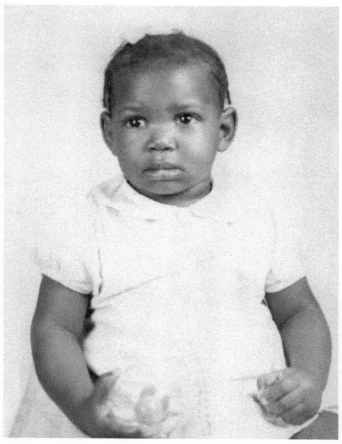

Deanna Midgette, 1945.

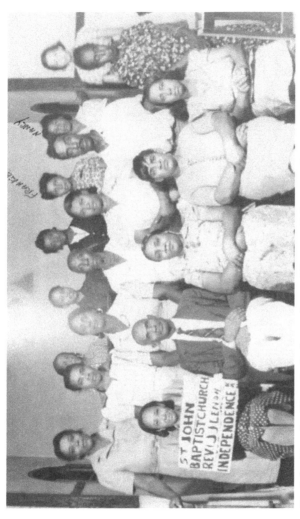

St. John Baptist Church, Independence, Kansas, July 1941, Reverend J.J. Lenon, Pastor – the church Mama and Aunt Nancy grew up in and sang in the choir. Also this was the church where Mama played the piano.

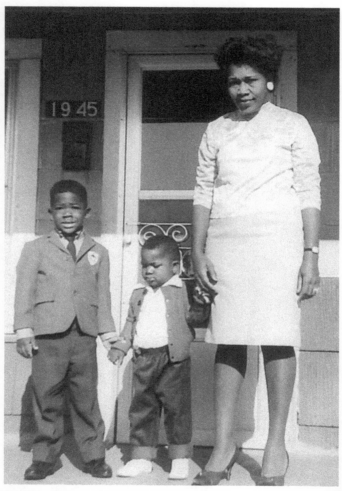

The Bruners 1964.

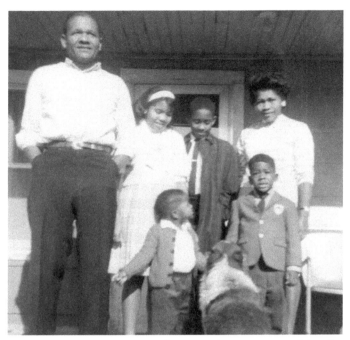

The Bruners 1964: Sam, Elaine, Brian, Larry, Michael, Frankie, and our dog Friskie.

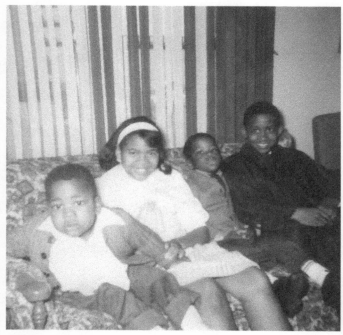

The Bruners 1964.

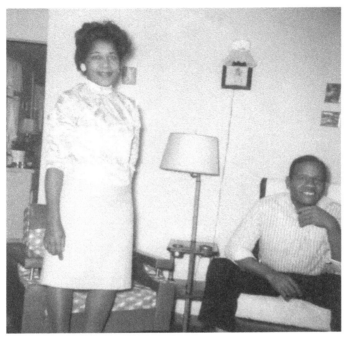

The Bruners 1964.

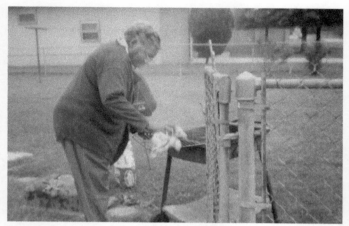

Mama firing up the grill.

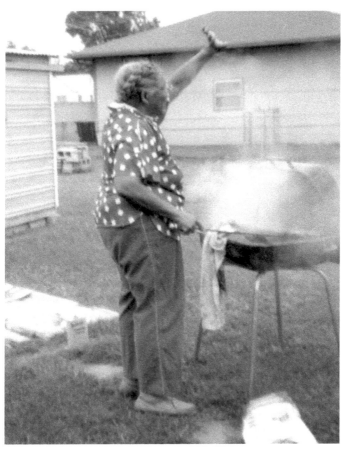

One of Mama's favorite things is outdoor barbecuing.
Her home, located on the corner, attracts many people
walking or driving by. As cars pass by they blew their
horns and Mama gave them a wave.

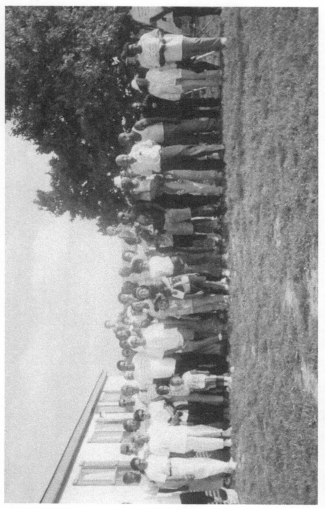

Smith-Bruner Family Reunion, May 27, 1994.

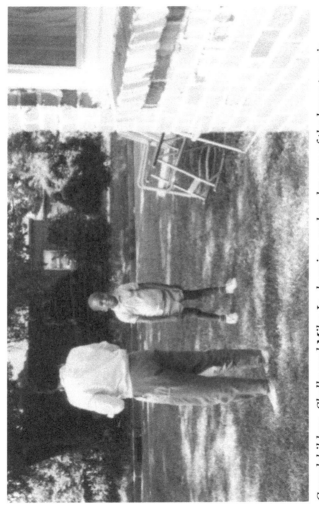

Grandchildren, Shelly and Mike Jr., keeping cool under one of the large trees in the yard.

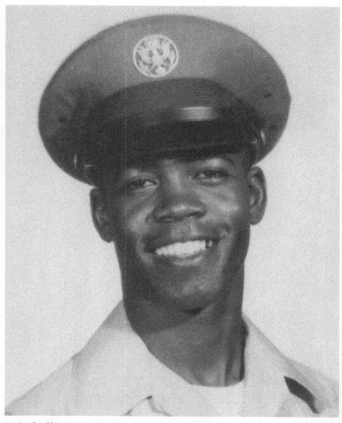

Mitchell B.

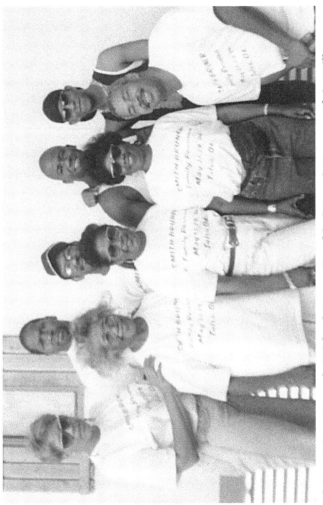

Elaine, Brian, Kenneth, Michael, Larry, Frankie (Mama), Deanna, Elois, Wilbert.

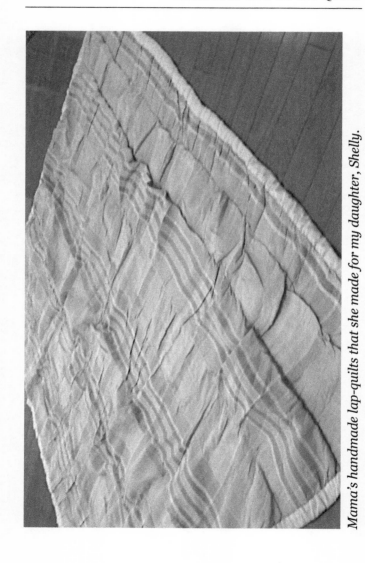

Mama's handmade lap-quilts that she made for my daughter, Shelly.

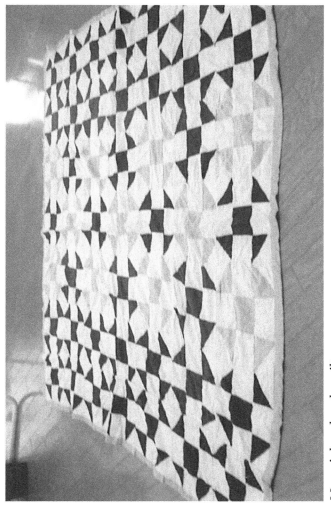

Mama's handmade quilt.

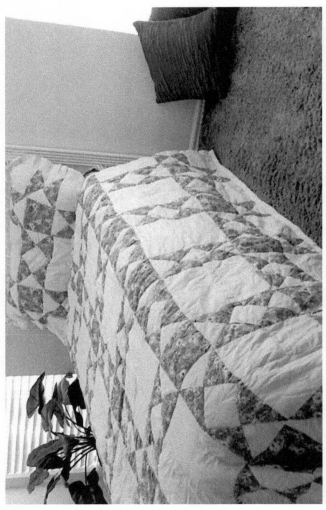

Mama hand-made this twin bed quilt and sham for me.

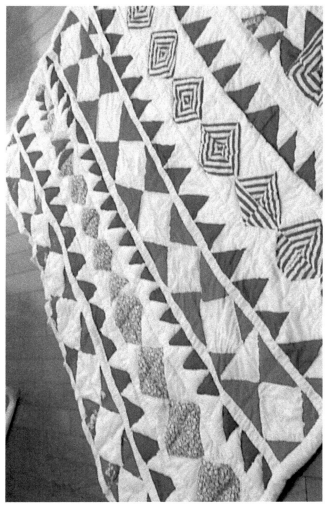

This is my first handmade quilt that Mama taught me when we had our quilting club.

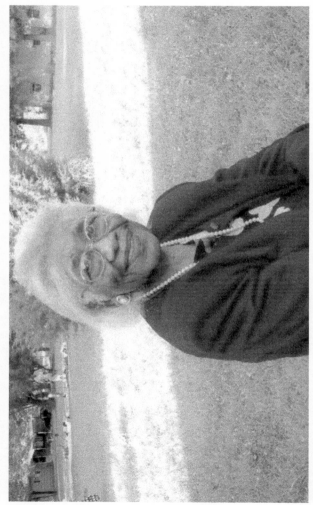

Frankie Bruner, 84 years of age, Independence, Kansas Homecoming Reunion, July 8, 2004.

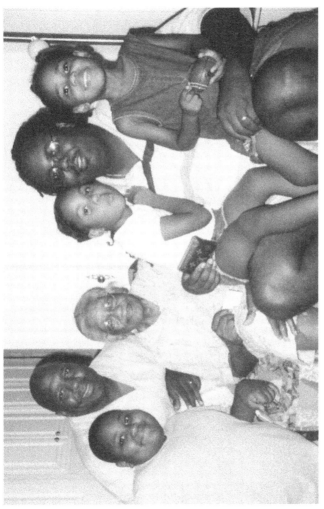

Grandma Frankie with grandchildren and great-grandchildren.

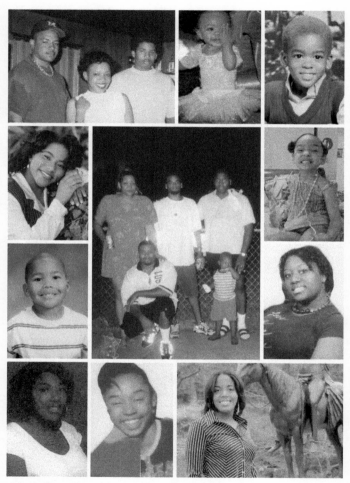

Grandma Frankie's grandchildren and great-grandchildren.

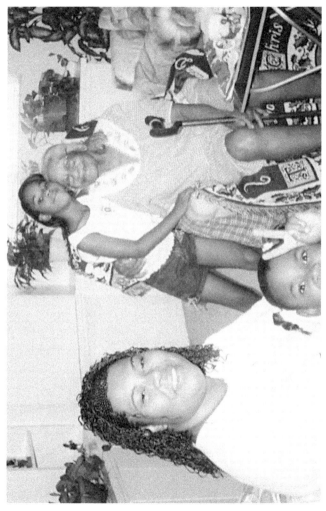

Grandma Frankie with grandchildren and great-grandchildren.

The Quilting Club

Hand-quilting, also called lap-quilting, was a hobby Mama truly loved. Mama's quilts were usually the size of a twin bedspread, which was just right for throwing across your body while watching television or for toddlers to lie on.

When I moved Mama from her home, I boxed up all of the scrap material she used for quilts, because I thought quilting would surely keep her busy. It did. In fact, she taught my friend and me how to quilt during her time with me. Mama's routine every morning would be to make her bed, wash, have breakfast, and work on her quilt. She would quilt from morning until evening, or until she got tired.

Mama made quilts for all of her children, and I still have the one she made for me. Mama seldom kept her own quilts. She usually gave them to family and friends. If she was working on a quilt, she would ask, "Did I ever make you a quilt?" If the answer was no, she would say, "Well, this quilt is yours." But you would have to watch that quilt because as she got older and her memory became short, you might not get your quilt, but you could be sure someone else would come along and claim it.

However, one morning, something was different. As I went about my morning routine, I noticed that she was unusually quiet, so I checked on her. When I entered her room, she was sitting in her rocking chair crying and saying, "Someone cut up my quilt!" When I saw the cut pieces of material on the floor, I asked her, "Did you do that?" She said, "NO!" I quickly defended myself and said, "I didn't do it!" I thought to myself, "Why would anyone want to play a horrible joke on her? Who would grab a pair of scissors and start hacking and slicing on other people's work?" I was amazed and shocked as I picked up the pieces of material and examined the quilt. There were squares cut out of the center of the quilt, as if someone were trying to cut more squares for another quilt. I thought, "Who could have done this evil thing?" I settled Mama down, and then we tried to figure out how to piece the quilt back together. But the same thing happened again the next day. The same quilt we pieced and sewed back together was cut again during the night. I wasn't that naive. I began to suspect she was cutting her own quilts. But I was unable to prove it. I would stay up late at night to try and catch her in the act, but it never happened.

Only two other people were living in the home besides me: my husband, Madison, and my daughter, Shelly, and neither cared anything about her quilts. I speculated she would wait until everyone was asleep and silently massacre the quilt. After patiently sewing the pieces back together a third time, I knew this would not stop; therefore, I hid the quilt and did not encourage her to start a new one.

A few weeks later, as I was thinking of something for her to do, I thought it would be a great idea if she could teach my friend and me how to quilt. She liked that idea, and as we'd sat on the floor, Mama, sitting in her favorite chair, happily gave us instructions. It was a lot of fun. We had our own quilting club!

The quilting club was not without drama

though. One morning as we sat on the floor with our quilts, ready to start sewing, Mama became agitated and accused us of stealing her quilt. She said, "Where is my quilt? I had one just like that!" And so, the quilting club ended. But we did eventually complete our quilts, and I am thankful to Mama for inspiring us to learn.

Today, I sometimes pull out the quilts and fondly remember our quilting club.

———

"To everything there is a season, and a time to every purpose under the heaven: A time to rend, and a time to sew; a time to keep silence, and a time to speak;" (Ecclesiastes 3:1,7).

The Grocery Store

Going to the grocery store with Mama was also a memorable experience. Again, I always kept her wheelchair in my car just in case she became tired of walking when we'd go out. Once, I decided to take her wheelchair into the grocery store so she could sit in it while I did the shopping.

I grabbed a grocery cart and left Mama sitting in an area where I could watch her. I picked up a few canned goods and returned to the spot where I had left her, and she was still sitting there. I thought, "Great, I'll go and get some more items." I told her I needed one more item, and I would be right back. But when I returned, she was gone and the wheelchair was empty. Mama was nowhere in sight. I put my shopping cart back, grabbed her wheelchair, put my groceries in the wheelchair, and began searching for her.

I finally found her walking around and scared because she thought I had left her. I got her into the wheelchair and pushed her around while she held the groceries in her lap. At the checkout counter, while I was putting groceries on the conveyor belt, Mama jumped out of the wheelchair and said, "I don't need that wheelchair! I can walk!" Then she walked away. I was yelling, "Mama! Let me check out first. Wait! Don't go anywhere!" As I put my grocery bags in the wheelchair and walked out the door, I started singing to myself, "No more trips to the grocery store!"

―――――

"Speaking to yourselves in psalms and hymns and spiritual songs, singing and making melody in your heart to the Lord;"
(Ephesians 5:19).

The Eating Patterns

Mama's eating patterns became a complex issue. I would make breakfast, and she would eat it. I would prepare lunch, and she'd eat that. When my daughter or husband ate a late lunch or snack, she would tell them she had not eaten all day. Mama would eat and snack with everyone in the house.

I began to take note of the times when she said she was hungry. She became hungry about every four hours. I learned to give her a snack between meals and a snack before bedtime, when necessary.

But there were days Mama would not want to eat at all, and she would make excuses for not eating. Her excuses would be, "I never eat a big meal." Or she'd say, "It's too salty," or "It's too hot."

The great lesson I learned was to pray before trying to command, plead, beg, or advise Mama to do anything or go anywhere. *"Evening, and morning, and at noon, will I pray, and cry aloud; and he shall hear my voice." (Psalms 55:17)*

Eventually, I found keywords to get her to eat. I had to use the word *coffee* in the place of the word *breakfast* because when I asked Mama if she wanted breakfast, her answer would be, *"No, I never eat breakfast, I only eat a piece of toast and drink a cup of coffee."* But, when I asked if she wanted *coffee,* she would eat whatever I put in front of her.

Mama loved diet Dr. Pepper, but I had to remove that from her diet because she could drink three or four in one day, so I substituted Hawaiian Punch in the can. I feared she would develop a urinary infection from the soda pop. Sometimes she'd ask for that "strong drink," and I knew the drink she was referring to, but I also knew better than to answer her. I didn't want to start that addiction up again. It was goodbye Dr. Pepper!

Mama had a fancy for Kleenex, napkins, and paper towels. Her hands always felt sweaty, and she needed to wipe them often. She would fold every napkin or paper towel given to her and place them in her purse. I would find paper products stacked in the dresser drawers, sometimes with money and food wrapped up in them. The food Mama would wrap were mostly meats that were difficult to chew or she got tired of chewing on. She'd wrap up pieces of candy, cake, and cookies. She would also wrap her medication up, and I'd find them in her purse and dresser, which meant a daily check of her purse and dresser drawers. I usually did the checking during the day, when she was not in her room, following the scripture, *I Corinthians 14:40, "Let all things be done decently and in order."* Meaning, when she was not watching!

Hygiene

Every morning Mama would get dressed, make her bed, wash her face, and brush her teeth with no problem. As time went on, however, I noticed Mama had stopped changing her clothes. She would put on the same clothing as the day before, which was usually not soiled.

At home, Mama liked to wear dusters that zipped, snapped, or buttoned up the front. They were comfortable and easy to put on and take off. She wore whole slips under her dusters to eliminate the need to wear a bra. She also wore incontinence panties that were 100 percent cotton for protection. Mama loved to wear knee high stockings with her tennis shoes, but the stockings became too tight around her calves; therefore, I would buy pantyhose and cut the legs off and twist them loosely above the knees.

Later, I had to switch out the tennis shoes for support shoes without shoe strings. She could just slip them on and off, and they were great for all types of weather and any occasion.

Mama always washed and pressed her own hair, until I noticed she was burning her skin with the hot iron. I also noticed that she would fall asleep in the middle of pressing her hair. That scared me! I would ask her if I could help her, and she would immediately lecture me: She was a professional beautician and could do her own hair. Then I would say to her, "Well, if you don't let me practice on your hair, how can I learn what you taught me about washing and pressing hair. I need someone to practice on." Then Mama would stop fussing and say, "Well, I guess you will have to practice on me." From then on, I did not have to worry about her burning herself or burning my house down.

Did I enjoy "washing hair day?" It could have been fun, were it not for the same lecture I got from Mama each time about being a *professional beautician* and being able to do her own hair. And EACH TIME, I would have to repeat my lines, "But who will I practice on?" It was not unusual for Mama to comb her hair three to six times a day. If I combed her hair after her shower, she would take it down and comb it again several times throughout the day. But as Alzheimer's slowly set in, Mama stopped combing her hair.

Hygiene was an area I thought could be administered without any problems, but as the Alzheimer's progressed, I was wrong. Mama began to refuse to bathe or shower. I thought, maybe she did not want me, her daughter, looking at her nude body and giving her instructions on bathing. After questioning Mama about not changing clothes and refusing to take baths or showers, her answer was, "The doctor instructed me not to take baths or showers." But I sympathized with her, because I feared she would fall getting in and out of the tub and shower. I installed handrails and a shower seat for her safety, but she still refused to let me assist her in taking baths. A woman from our church agreed to come in once a week to help me with Mama. She was truly God-sent. She even found keywords to use for Mama's bath time. Instead of saying bath or shower, the keywords were, *"Let's take a wash off."* She also believed in prayer and prayed before helping Mama.

Bath days also could be challenging. I called these days a test of the *long-suffering*. On bath days, there was usually the *bad person* who got her up to bathe and the good person who gave her the bath. Of course, I was the bad person. On bath days, I usually awakened Mama at least 10 minutes before the caregiver arrived. If Mama started asking questions such as: "Why are you waking me up? Why do I have to take a wash off? Where am I going?" Or, she said, "I'm already dressed!" Then I knew this was going to be a *long-suffering day*. It was around the time when the caregiver was usually walking into the room, and Mama saw her as the *good person!* Mama would say, "Hi honey, I'm so glad to see you," and that would be my cue to leave the room.

Then there were days when Mama did not recognize the caregiver, and the caregiver would sit down on the bed and talk with Mama a few minutes. Soon after, I would hear them laughing, and then I'd hear the water in the shower running. I thank God for the small things.

———

"A merry heart maketh a cheerful countenance: ..." (Proverbs 15:13).

Running away

While we were still living in Peoria, Arizona, in 2003, I left Mama in my daughter's care while I went to church. Mama, thinking she was at work, decided she wanted to *quit her job* and leave the house. When my daughter tried to persuade her back into the house, she raised her walking cane and threatened to strike her with it.

When I arrived home, Mama was across the street telling our neighbors, "I quit cleaning house for that person who lives across the street because that woman has a gun and tried to shoot me." (A tip that I learned from this incident: Any information from an Alzheimer's patient can be blown out of proportion, so always check the facts.) Of course, our neighbors were quite shaken up after hearing Mama's story and actually called the police. However, everything was explained to the police, they understood, and we all settled down again.

But that was not the only incident involving Mama and the police.

In 2006, after moving to Edmond, Oklahoma, Mama would usually stay with her niece Elaine at her house when I traveled. Ernest Jr., Elaine's son, was watching Mama while staying at the house one evening. While Ernest watched television, Mama got up and left the room. He assumed she was headed to the bathroom, but she instead headed out the front door. Mama noticed Elaine's neighbors were outside talking in their yard, and she decided to cross the street. She told them she had been kidnapped and asked the startled neighbors to call the police. After the police were called, Mama told the dispatcher on the phone that she had been kidnapped. The dispatcher then became confused when Mama provided her Tulsa address as her current location. Meanwhile, after realizing she was gone, my cousin went outside to look for Mama and saw her with the neighbors. Ernest spoke with the dispatcher and was able to convince the dispatcher that his aunt had dementia and was not kidnapped, and the police did not need to rush to the scene. Today, my cousin still talks about that incident.

———

"A SOFT answer turneth away wrath: ..."
(Proverbs 15:1).

Canes vs. Walkers

Mama was not a big television watcher, but she did like to watch certain daytime shows. I had to monitor what she was watching, because Mama would think that the actors on the television show were real, and if she were in an argumentative mood, she would talk back.

The reality of her reactions to television was among the reasons I had to replace Mama's walking cane with a walker to avoid harm to her and others. When she was grumpy or thought she might be harmed, she used her walking cane as a weapon. She would raise it to hit or scare people away. And she actually raised her walking cane to hit the actors on the television show. Thus, the switch from cane to *walker* prevented a broken television screen. At first, the transition did not go well, but slowly she became used to the walker. It proved to be a great choice for her because it gave her more stability than the walking cane, and it provided safety for everyone else – and my television.

Once I heard Mama talking to the television and telling the actors on the show to leave her *walker* alone. When I heard her arguing, I went to look in on her and saw her walker had been placed in front of the television. She was accusing the actors in the show of stealing her walker. I decided to move the walker and place it next to her chair; that ended the argument. After that when Mama became upset while watching television, I usually turned to the Christian channel, and she'd fall asleep.

———

"When thou liest down, thou shalt not be afraid; yea, thou shalt lie down, and thy sleep shall be sweet." (Proverbs 3:24).

Going Home

When we had visitors to the home, Mama would sit by them and speak very softly to ask for a ride home; however, she only did that with people she knew from Tulsa. But when they were leaving, she never made any effort to go with them. She would say goodbye and act as if she had never asked them for a ride home.

Some days, Mama would want to go home to Kansas, and she would continue to say over and over again, "I want to go home." She would pretend to be sick and ask me to call a doctor. She would *fake cry* (crying without tears) and speak in a little girl's voice as if mocking a little child.

It was then that I would call Elaine. She was my relief caregiver, and Mama would spend a few days with Elaine and her husband, Ernest. Those were great breaks for Mama -- and for me. *"... Separate thyself ..." (Genesis 13: 9).*

Sundown Arguments

At dinnertime, Mama would start arguments.

"I don't like this; it's too hot," or "You shouldn't feed kids this hot food," she'd say.

I'd reply sarcastically, "That food is not hot."

The argument would intensify.

She'd then yell, "I'm going home to get my own dinner!"

"You can't go home by yourself," I'd reply.

"I'll call the police on you!" When she asked for the telephone, I'd give her a television remote control from another room. If she look puzzled, I would say, "Try again later, they are probably out of the office."

In the evening, as the sun began to set, Mama went through her routine of *getting home before dark*. This was repeated every night. After dinner, she would say, "Get the little boys, and let's go home." "The little boys" she was referring to were my two youngest brothers, Michael and Brian. She would tell us to call her dad or her brothers to pick her up because her mother was waiting for her. Then she would walk back and forth, from room to room, until she was exhausted. After her legs became weak from walking, she'd finally go to bed.

As I made my rounds each night, checking her room to make sure she had water, the blinds were closed, and the night light was on in the bathroom, the strangest, most phenomenal thing would happen almost every night. She would smile and say, "Thanks for taking care of me. You are a sweet girl. See you in the morning."

When I heard those words, I'd think to myself, "I've been entertaining an angel unaware; where did that person come from?" I have heard that words of kindness are like glittering diamonds. Then the eventful day ends, and I would get up the next morning to repeat the same ritual again, day after day. *"And David was greatly distressed ... but David encouraged himself in the Lord his God." (I Samuel 30:6)*. Each day I put to practice these powerful words to encourage myself as a caregiver.

Mama's Late Stages

"Today, my mother was giving me her jew-elry, some small change, a scarf, etc. She asked me, 'Did I give this to you?' ... Or 'Here take this, I want you to have this.' And I would politely say okay. Later, I realized she was putting her last possessions in my hands! My daughter, Shelly, mentioned to me that Grandma was saying, 'Jesus is coming.' My husband, Madi-son, also noticed how she was singing 'all the hymns she knew.' "

That is what I wrote in my journal on May 3, 2009, as Mama's condition worsened.

Then in September the same year, I prayed, "God help me make the best decision for Mama." At this point, she was not walking or talking, and unable to get herself out of bed. Mama had made frequent trips to the hospital for dehydra-tion, because she was not eating and not getting enough fluids. I was told I would have to admit her into a nursing home or look into hospice-at-home. My relatives, Kenneth, Brian, Anne, and

I, decided to check out nursing facilities, but we did not want her in a nursing home. However, we checked out the options. I prayed, "God, I don't want her to go to a nursing facility; please give me direction with peace of mind." I knew I would spend more time going back and forth to the nursing home, making sure she was comfortable and eating. I wondered to myself: Who would be there for her when I was worn out physically and mentally? Or, what if the weather was bad, and I was unable to see her?

I reflected on the questions as I read the book *Coach Broyles' Playbook for Alzheimer's Caregivers* by Frank Broyles, former athletic director for the University of Arkansas. Broyles wrote about the decisions he faced in caring for his wife, Barbara, who suffered from Alzheimer's:

> *"Many caregivers make the choice to move their loved one into a nursing home during this stage. Your daily visits and love is the key to getting good care for your loved ones in the nursing home. Get to know the*

staff and help them get to know your loved one. Now is the time for caregivers to take care of themselves. Remember to celebrate the smallest successes. Allow yourself to grieve your loss. Give your body time to regain strength. Take care of your own health." [3]

My decision soon became clear, and I decided to do hospice-at-home. Mercy Hospital Oklahoma City, where Mama had already been admitted, had a hospice-at-home program. After being evaluated, she qualified to be under hospice care, and the arrangements were made to keep her at home.

Mama's health steadily declined, and I notified my family that her days were short. On Sunday, November 1, 2009, everyone was at the house, and my brother Larry, who lived in Sacramento, California, called on the phone. Everyone talked to her and told her what she had meant to them as a mother, and they told her that they would be well and not to worry about them. After seeing her children, I believe this gave Mama the release she needed to pass over.

On the night of November 3, 2009, Shelly and I were in her room talking when Mike Jr., my nephew, called and said he was in town and on his way to the house. For some reason, I believe Mama heard my conversation on the telephone, and it was as if her spirit went to the door with me to greet him. When Mike and I walked into her bedroom, her eyes were fixed, and we all knew she'd passed on from this life into eternity.

On November 21, 2009, I wrote this in my journal:

"Mom's journey ended on Nov. 3, 2009 at 9:30 p.m. Tuesday night. My nephew, Mike Jr. called. He arrived in Oklahoma City and was on his way over to the house. As he rang the doorbell, Mama closed her eyes at the age of 89 years, and went home with the Lord Jesus."

I believe the meaning of death is described best in the *Journal of Religious*.

Gerontology 7:

*"According to logotherapy, our own past
is our true future. While we are alive, we
have both a future and a past; the dying
man has no future in the usual sense, but
only a past; the dead, however, 'is' his past.
He has no life, he 'is' his life. We become a
reality, not at our birth, but rather at our
death. Our self 'is' not something that 'is'
but something that is becoming, and therefore becomes itself fully only when life has
been completed by death. We are 'creating'
ourselves at the moment of our death."* 4

After her life ended on earth, I chose to remember the mother who rubbed my legs daily
when I suffered from polio, who never gave up
on herself or her children, who accepted others
with a friendly wave or a place for them to sleep
at night, who cooked delicious meals and left her
recipes for all of us to enjoy, who created beautiful quilts that will live beyond her earthly body,
and who left a family who will love her always.
To everyone, she was our Mama. My sacrifice

toward the end of her life could never replace her sacrifice at the beginning of mine and my brothers and sisters.

As I reminisce about my time with Mama during her illness, I found *four basic attitudes* that kept my focus: being prayerful, patient, respectful, and NEVER getting drawn into an argument. My advice to you is simple: Do everything you can to make your loved ones feel special. At the end of the day, REJOICE that you both survived -- to be repeated again! The Bible verse that ends this book is the reason for my belief that Mama and I will be together again someday. I hope it provides you with the same hope if you're going through what I did with Mama: *"For God so loved the world, that He gave his only begotten Son, that whosoever believeth in him should not perish, but have everlasting life." (John 3:16).*

Epilogue

I wrote this poem when the Lord Jesus compelled me to look back on those moments when my mother and I could laugh together.   She would call me Mama Lois, and I would call her Miss Frankie.

Mama Lois and Miss Frankie

The day will come
when I will live with you,
like you lived with me.
I ask that you have patience,
and understanding of the things I do.
When I'm an old lady
and my memory is short,
please remember these moments,
for your time is also becoming short.

Don't get angry
when I draw on the wall,
and scuff up your floor,
with my walker in one hand
and my cane you hung on the door.

When crumbs fall on the floor,
don't mumble under your breath,
just get the broom and remember
how I cleaned up your mess.

When I ask for my mom and dad
and you tell me they're dead,
I'll ask you to prove it,
because those were the best days I had.
If you correct me, I'll lie down
and cry, kicking and screaming,
not a tear in my eye.

If I repeat the same things over
and over again, don't interrupt and say,
"I've heard that before!"
A wise one would listen and learn to discern,
how to be patient with the chattering,
for they are only words,
not knowing how to end.

If I hide my glasses in my sock,
and put my food inside my drawer,
don't scold me too bad,
because I'll just hang my head,

and in a moment not remember
what had been said.

As long as you are busy,
I won't leave you alone, I'll pester you
when I think you're on the phone.
If I don't want a shower or bath,
especially given by you, remember,
I'm still the parent and not used
to my nudeness in front of you.

When I pull out my clothes,
but forget how to dress,
notice when I pull out my red coat,
that means take me home, I need my rest.

– AUTHOR, ELOIS MIDGETTE CAMPBELL

Resources

1 The Independence, KS, Homecoming Reunions, *A Preview of Independence, KS African-American History* by Bennie Jr. and Charlene Mosely: Chapter 7: History of African-American Contractors/ Builders, pg. 79-80.

2 Master's Graduate School of Divinity, Course Title: *Gerontology Cassette #4,* Riseburg Model: Course Assessor: Matthew Crandall, Evansville: 2002.

3 Broyles, J. Frank, Coach Broyles' *Playbook for Alzheimer's Caregivers,* the University of Arkansas of Trustees, 2006.

4 Seeber, James J., *Journal of Religious Gerontology 7,* New York: The Haworth Press Inc., 1990.

Other References

Books:

Clements, Williams M., *Ministry with the Aging,*
Binghamton: The Haworth Press, Inc., 1989.

Survival Kit for Seniors, Oklahoma City:
Areawide Aging Agency, Inc.
Senior Connection, 3200 NW 48th Street, Suite 105
Oklahoma City, OK 73112
405-943-4344

Support Group:

Alzheimer's Association
Oklahoma Support Group Meetings
1-800-272-3900
www.Alz.org

Legal Service:

Legal Services for the Elderly Hotline
1-800-750-5353

Hospice:

Mercy Hospice Oklahoma City
405-752-3590

Appendix 1

What is Alzheimer's?

In a Master's graduate course, *Gerontology Studies,* I learned that Alzheimer's has seven stages, according to the *Riseburg Model:* [2]

Stages 1-3 are rarely or almost undetectable.

Stage 4 is the late confusion stage: This is the point where the indications of dementia are becoming observable.   If the person is still at home, most people are unaware of their developing patterns.

Stage 5 is early dementia (all dressed-up with no place to go): The person looks normal. They get up make their bed, and put on their clothes. They still wear jewelry, make-up, glasses, their speech is good, and immediate memory is still intact. However, their short memory may not recall your visit the day before, and they may not be able to tell you what they had for breakfast or remember taking their medication. Stage 5 will take them back in time looking for those responsibilities they had at a younger age. They don't believe they need assistance. They will seek to leave, run away, or start to go somewhere and lose their train of thought.

Stage 6 is mild dementia ("I want to go with you."): They will latch on to someone they frequently see and want to go with them everywhere or get a ride home. This is a fear of being left alone. They will not change their clothing if you don't give them clothes to change into. They will put on the same soiled and dirty clothing that they wore the day before. A change of clothing is new clothing to them; also, at this stage, they will stop wearing make-up and jewelry, because they'll get tired of putting it on. Women will stop carrying their purses, wearing glasses, pantyhose, or whatever is a support to them. They will go along with sex, but they do not have a real sex drive. Some do not like taking showers, but will take a bath or the reversal, take a bath, but will not shower.

Stage 7 is last stage of Alzheimer's (no ability): Their physical appearance is abnormal. They don't look right by our normal social standard. They fiddle with their clothes, wear a sweatsuit in the summer, and short sleeves in the cold winter. They have a tendency to take off shoes and socks. They will not carry on a conversation with you. They will sit and stare. You have to persuade them to eat. They often mistake a shower chair or wastebasket as a toilet seat. This is the time you will need to address them by their first name. There will be a period of weight loss. They have no knowledge of being human. At this time they will lose their ability to move around, sit up, hold their head up to swallow -- and death soon follows. Spiritual support is extremely important. Caregivers should be encouraged to use hospice and other services in their community and take some time to recover themselves from the extreme stress and anxiety of being a caregiver.

Appendix 2

List of My Supported Scriptures as a Caregiver.
All Scripture quotations are from the King
James Bible (KJV)

1. Abiding in the Vine ....John 15

Verse 4: Abide in me, and I in you. As the branch cannot bear fruit of itself, except it abide in the vine; no more can ye, except ye abide in me.

Verse 5: I am the vine, ye are the branches: He that abideth in me, and I in him, the same bringeth forth much fruit: for without me ye can do nothing.

2. Love Chapter............................... I Corinthians 13

Verses 4-8: Charity (love) suffereth long, and is kind; charity envieth not; charity vaunteth not itself, is not puffed up, Doth not behave itself unseemly, seeketh not her own, is not easily

*provoked, thinketh no evil; Rejoiceth not in
iniquity, but rejoiceth in the truth; Beareth all
things, believeth all things, hopeth all things,
endureth all things. Charity never faileth: but
whether there be prophecies, they shall fail;
whether there be tongues, they shall cease;
whether there be knowledge, it shall vanish away.*

3. Consecration Chapter .... Romans 12

*Verses 12-15: Rejoicing in hope; patient in
tribulation; continuing instant in prayer;
Distributing to the necessity of saints; given to
hospitality. Bless them which persecute you; bless,
and curse not. Rejoice with them that do rejoice,
and weep with them that weep.*

4. Faith Chapter .... Hebrews 11

*Verse 6: But without faith it is impossible to please
him: for he that cometh to God must believe that he*

is, and that he is a rewarder of them that diligently seek him.

5. Heaven Chapter .... Revelation 21

Verse 1: And I saw a new heaven and a new earth: for the first heaven and the first earth were passed away; and there was no more sea.

Verse 4: And God shall wipe away all tears from their eyes; and there shall be no more death, neither sorrow, nor crying, neither shall there be any more pain: for the former things are passed away.

6. Holy Spirit Chapter.....................................John 16

Verse 13: Howbeit when he, the Spirit of truth, is come, he will guide you into all truth: for he shall not speak of himself; but whatsoever he shall hear, that shall he speak: and he will shew you things to come.

7. Prayer Chapter .... John 17

*Verses 1-5: These words spake Jesus, and lifted
up his eyes to heaven, and said, Father, the hour
is come; glorify thy Son, that thy Son also may
glorify thee: As thou hast given him power over all
flesh, that he should give eternal life to as many as
thou hast given him. And this is life eternal, that
they might know thee the only true God, and Jesus
Christ, whom thou hast sent. I have glorified thee
on the earth: I have finished the work which thou
gavest me to do. And now, O Father, glorify thou
me with thine own self with the glory which I had
with thee before the world was.*

8. Marriage Chapter .... Ephesians 5

*Verses 21-22: Submitting yourselves one to
another in the fear of God. Wives, submit
yourselves unto your own husbands, as unto the
Lord.*

Verse 25: Husbands, love your wives, even as Christ also loved the church, and gave himself for it;

Verse 28: So ought men to love their own bodies. He that loveth his wife loveth himself.

Verse 31: For this cause shall a man leave his father and mother, and shall be joined unto his wife, and they two shall be one flesh.

9. Peace Chapter ....John 14

Verse 27: Peace I leave with you, my peace I give unto you: not as the world giveth, give I unto you. Let not your heart be troubled, neither let it be afraid.

10. Victory Chapter ....Romans 8

Verse 27: And he that searcheth the hearts knoweth what is the mind of the Spirit, because he maketh intercession for the saints according to the will of God.

Verse 28: And we know that all things work together for good to them that love God, to them who are the called according to his purpose.

Appendix 3

Medical Information Form
Sample Copy

Year:

Patient Name:

Date of Birth:

Allergic To:

Blood Type:

Surgery or Hospitalized: (list type and year)

1.

2.

3.

Test Procedures & Physical Exam (list date)

1.

2.

3.

4.

Specialist:

1.

2.

3.

Other Procedures & Shots:

1.

2.

3.

Medications: (list mg. dosage, Xdaily)

1.

2.

3.

Weight: _____ Height: _____

Last Follow-Up: _____ Next Visit: _____

Appendix 4

Elois's Personal Checklist for Caregiver

Alert Signs:

1. Watch for complaints of continually forgetting location of objects, (e.g., keys, purse, eyeglasses).

2. Beware of accusations that you, family members, friends and strangers are stealing from them. (e.g., money, keys, jewelry, purse).

3. Watch for their decreased ability to perform complex tasks (e.g., handling personal finances, falling asleep while cooking, forgetting how to plan dinner, not paying bills).

4. Loved ones may require assistance in choosing proper clothing to wear for the day (e.g. they may wear the same clothing repeatedly, if not supervised).

5. Watch loved one's personal hygiene -- they may be

unable to bathe properly (e.g., difficulty with water temperature, afraid of baths and showers, getting in and out of closed spaces, fearful of falling).

Taking over a Loved One's Affairs:

1. Obtain durable power of attorney for health and financial management. This should be done while parents or loved ones are still independent.

2. Retrieve personal papers (e.g., birth records, marriage and divorce records, Social Security card, Medicare or Medicaid card).

3. Retrieve insurance papers (e.g., life and burial, home, car, Medicare supplement, Medicare part D medicine plan, long-term care insurance).

4. Make an appointment with a doctor to get proper diagnosis and physical examination. (Always go into the exam room with your loved ones. They may not understand what the doctors are saying.)

5. Take notes of office visits and keep a list of all medications. (This will be helpful in the days and years to come.)

6. Start considering housing (e.g., residential care, assisted living, keeping parents or loved ones in your own home, or move in with them).

7. Take time to check out adult daycare centers and support groups for yourself.

8. All caregivers should take time to meditate or try another form of relaxation.

About the Author

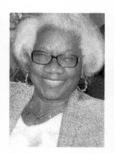

Elois Midgette Campbell was born in Tulsa, Oklahoma. She has lived in Omaha, Nebraska, Oakland, California, Phoenix, Arizona, and now in Edmond, Oklahoma, with her husband of 38 years, Madison Campbell. After 21 years of service, she retired from the federal government's Department of Energy as an Engineering Technician in Phoenix.

Elois served four years as a Bible instructor for the Manhattan Bible Institute West in Phoenix. She has traveled to Haiti with the Equator Faith Mission World Outreach Ministries as a missionary. She has taught Bible studies in her home, adopted a Bible study/ prayer group for a women's homeless shelter, and served as assistant chapter leader for the Christian Women's Devotional Alliance (CWDA) in the Glendale/ Peoria, Arizona, area. She enjoys working in the various auxiliaries of her church, Victory Temple Church of God in Christ, in Oklahoma City, and monthly nursing home visitation.

Elois has earned an Associate Degree of General Studies (AGS), a Bachelor Degree of Religious Education (BRE), and a Master of Ministry Degree (MM) in Biblical Counseling.

Her favorite Scriptures are many, but Psalms 23 has carried her throughout life.

Her Mission Statement: When you find people who are hungry for learning, teach them all that you can.

CPSIA information can be obtained
at www.ICGtesting.com
Printed in the USA
FFHW021417050619
52848493-58397FF